QuickPath

A Pathology Quick guide for Massage Therapist & other Professionals

PARKER MASER

QuickPath © Copyright 2025 Parker Maser

All rights reserved. No part of this publication may be reproduced, distributed or transmitted in any form or by any means, including photocopying, recording, or other electronic or mechanical methods, without the prior written permission of the publisher, except in the case of brief quotations embodied in critical reviews & certain other noncommercial uses permitted by copyright law.

Although the author & publisher have made every effort to ensure that the information in this book was correct at press time, the author & publisher do not assume & hereby disclaim any liability to any party for any loss, damage, or disruption caused by errors or omissions, whether such errors or omissions result from negligence, accident, or any other cause.

Adherence to all applicable laws & regulations, including international, federal, state & local governing professional licensing, business practices, advertising, & all other aspects of doing business in the US, Canada or any other jurisdiction is the sole responsibility of the reader & consumer.

Neither the author nor the publisher assumes any responsibility or liability whatsoever on behalf of the consumer or reader of this material. Any perceived slight of any individual or organization is purely unintentional.

The resources in this book are provided for informational purposes only & should not be used to replace the specialized training & professional judgment of a health care or mental health care professional.

Neither the author nor the publisher can be held responsible for the use of the information provided within this book. Please always consult a trained professional before making any decision regarding treatment of yourself or others.

ISBN: 979-8-89694-226-9 - Paperback
ISBN: 979-8-89694-225-2 - eBook

This book would not have been possible without the support, knowledge, and encouragement of so many incredible people.

To my classmates and fellow massage therapists—your time, insights, and willingness to help shape this project have been invaluable. Your dedication to this field continues to inspire me, and I am deeply grateful for the role you played in bringing *QuickPath* to life.

To the Spore Family, especially my best friend, Georgia Spore—thank you for always believing in me.

To my fellow massage therapists:

Stephanie Torres, Christian Florez-Castaneda, Shea Lozano, Amanda Latham, Jerico Celedonio, Mellissa Palmar, Alyssa Dimailig, & Yesica Leavy.

Artist: Gabriela Torres

Your contributions and passion for this profession have made a lasting impact.

To Zachary Maser, Kira Maser, and Julia Maser—your support has meant the world to me.

To my parents—thank you for your encouragement.

This book is as much yours as it is mine.

With gratitude,

Parker M

As massage therapists, we are constantly expanding our knowledge to better serve our clients. Understanding pathologies is a critical part of that journey—but too often, the information available is dense, complex, or buried in lengthy textbooks. That's why *QuickPath* was created.

This book is designed as a practical, easy-to-use reference for massage therapists who need quick, reliable information about various conditions they may encounter in practice. Whether you're reviewing a pathology before a session or refreshing your knowledge between clients, *QuickPath* provides concise, relevant details that help you make informed decisions about bodywork.

Each entry is written with clarity and simplicity, making even complex conditions easier to understand. By focusing on what truly matters in a massage therapy setting—contraindications, modifications, and key considerations—this book saves time while enhancing your ability to provide safe and effective care.

Massage therapy is not just about technique—it's about awareness, adaptability, and the ability to navigate the unique needs of each client. *QuickPath* is here to support you on that journey, offering a straightforward guide that empowers you to practice with confidence.

Welcome to *QuickPath*—your go-to resource for pathology insights in the massage therapy world.

Parker M
Author, Massage Therapist

KEY

R-pop - Regular Population

PN - Personal note

DT - Deep tissue

 -Contagious

 -Inflammatory

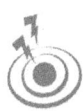 -Chronic pain/lifelong condition

MT - Massage Therapist

PT - Physical Therapist & Personal Trainer

PCP - Primary Care Physician

SHARP - Swelling, Hot, A Decreased ROM, Red, Pain

CONTENTS

A
Acne	13
Achilles Tendonosis	14
Acute Bronchitis	15
Adhesive Capsulitis (Frozen Shoulder)	16
ALS (Lou Gehrig Disease)	17
Alopecia Areata	18
Anemia	19
Ankylosing Spondylitis	20
Amplified Musculoskeletal Pain Syndrome (AMPS)	21
Arthritis	22
Anxiety	23
Asthma	24
Atherosclerosis	25

B
Baker's Cysts	26
Bell's Palsy	27
Bone Spurs	28
Bunions (Hallux Valgus)	29
Bursitis	30

C
Candidiasis	31
Carpal Tunnel Syndrome	32
Cellulitis	33
Cervical Palsy	34
Cervical Radiculopathy	35
Cirrhosis	36
Chronic Bronchitis	37
Chronic Pelvic Pain Syndrome	38
Compartment Disorder	39
Complex Regional Pain Syndrome(CRPS)	40
(COPD)Emphysema	41
Crohn's Disease	42

D

Diabetes Mellitus	43
Disc Disease	44
Dupuytren's Contracture (Palmar Fibromatosis)	45
Diverticular Disease	46
Dystonia	47

E

Eczema	48
Embolism (PE) & Thrombosis (DVT)	49
Encephalitis (West Nile Virus)	50
Ehlers-Danlos Syndrome	51
Endometriosis	52

F

Fibroid Tumors	53
Fibromyalgia	54

G

Gallstones	55
Ganglion Cysts	56
Gastroenteritis	57
Gout	58
Graves Disease	59

H

Hammertoe	60
Hepatitis(A,B & C)	61
Hernia	62
Herniated Disks	63
HIV/AIDS	64
Hives	65
Hyperkyphosis	66
Hypertension	67
Hypokyphosis	68
Hypothyroidism	69

I

Influenza	70
Irritable Bowel Syndrome(IBS)	71

J
Joint Replacement Surgery	72

K
Keloid Scars	73
Kidney Stones	74
Kidney Disease (Polycystic Kidney Disease, Pyelonephritis, & Renal Failure)	75

L
Lupus	76
Lyme Disease	77
Lymphedema	78
Lymphangitis	79

M
Metatarsalgia	80
Migraine Disorder	81
Mononucleosis	82
Morton's Neuroma	83
Multiple Sclerosis	84
Muscular Dystrophy	85

O
Osgood-Schlatter Disease	86
Osteoporosis(Porous Bones)	87
Osteoarthritis	88

P
Peripheral Neuropathy	89
Peptic Ulcer	90
Pes Planus, Pes Cavus (Flat & High arch foot)	91
Plantar Fasciitis	92
Pneumonia	93
Polycystic Kidney Disease	94
Postural Orthostatic Tachycardia Syndrome (POTS)	95
Prostatitis	96
Psoriasis	97
PTSD (Post Tramatic Stress Disorder)	98

R

Raynaud's Disease	99
Raynaud's Phenomenon	100
Rheumatoid Arthritis	101

S

Sever's Disease	102
Sciatica	103
Scleroderma (Systemic Sclerosis)	104
Seizure Disorders	105
Seborrheic Keratosis	106
Shin Splints (MTSS)	107
Sinusitis	108
Spondylolisthesis	109
Spinal Stenosis	110
Spondylosis	111
Sunburn	112

T

Tarsal Tunnel Syndrome	113
Tattoos (NEW)	114
Tennis Elbow & Golf Elbow	115
Tendinopathies	116
Temporomandibular Joint (TMJ)	117
Thoracic Outlet Syndrome	118
Tuberculosis	119

V

Vestibular Balance Disorders	120
Vitiligo	121

W

Warts	122
Whiplash	123

Z

Zoster (Shingles)	124
Understanding Medication	125
Treatment	127
Elderly Care (Parkinsons)	137
Understanding Supplement Benefits	139

ACNE

This is a common skin condition that occurs when pores become clogged with oil, dead skin cells, & sometimes bacteria. It most often appears on the face, chest, back, & shoulders. More common with teenagers, however, young adults can still have severe acne.

*PN-*Be mindful of hygiene when working on clients with active acne, especially if lesions are open or inflamed. Avoid applying excessive pressure over affected areas to prevent irritation or spread of bacteria.

Suggested Questions: Are you on any medications for your acne? Is your skin sensitive to any scented emollients?

Symptoms

- Clogged Pores (some may be red & cause pain if deep enough)
- Nodules-painful, solid lumps under the skin

Contraindications Local

- Gua sha
- Cupping
- Hot towels

ACHILLES TENDONOSIS

This is a chronic degeneration of the Achilles tendon due to overuse or improper healing. Clients with pronated feet are at a higher risk for this condition, which is typically caused by overuse. Rest is the most effective way to reduce pain & prevent further irritation.

*PN-*Clients may benefit from gentle myofascial work around the area but avoid deep pressure directly on the Achilles tendon. Ice therapy and stretching should only be done under medical guidance.

Suggested Questions: Has your PCP cleared you for massage? Are you working with a PT as well? Are you still currently playing sports, being active & staying on it?

Symptoms

- Pain & stiffness on the achilles
- Worsens with activity
- Burning & shooting pain in calves

Contraindications

- Deep tissue
- Heat
- Gua sha
- Active stretching

ACUTE BRONCHITIS

Inflammation of the bronchial tubes (airways) in the lungs, usually caused by a viral infection. Typically results in coughing, production of mucus, chest discomfort, & shortness of breath. Acute bronchitis often develops after a cold or respiratory infection. DO NOT MASSAGE clients until they have been cleared by PCP.

Symptoms

- Cough (w/mucus)
- Shortness of Breath
- Chest Discomfort
- Sore Throat
- Wheezing

Contraindication

- DO NOT MASSAGE

ADHESIVE CAPSULITIS (FROZEN SHOULDER)

"Frozen Shoulder" is when connective tissues that surround the glenohumeral joint (shoulder), becomes inflamed, thickened & restricted. Can last months or years but goes away on its own with time. In the first "Freezing" phase adhesive capsulitis may be painful & involve active inflammation.

PN-Massage can be beneficial in later phases to restore mobility, but avoid aggressive stretching or joint mobilization during the freezing and painful stages. Clients who have had a frozen shoulder on one side are more likely to get it on the other.

Suggested Questions: Are you currently taking any painkillers for your shoulder? How long have you been experiencing symptoms?

Symptoms

- Dull achy pain in shoulder
- Limited ROM
- Stiffness in joint

Contraindication Local

- Joint mobilization

ALS (LOU GEHRIG DISEASE)

Amyotrophic Lateral Sclerosis (ALS), also known as Lou Gehrig's Disease, is a progressive neurodegenerative disorder affecting nerve cells in the brain & spinal cord. This disease causes loss of muscle control & eventually leads to paralysis.

PN-DT is not needed for these clients; their muscles are already strained. Swedish technique should be used instead.

Symptoms

- Loss of muscle control in arms, legs, & neck.
- Trouble speaking
- Shortness of breath
- More prone to infections

Contraindication

- Deep Tissue

ALOPECIA AREATA

This is an autoimmune condition causing patchy hair loss on the scalp, face, & sometimes other areas of the body. Hair follicles are targeted by the immune system, leading to disrupted hair growth.

PN-Alopecia Areata can last for an extended period of time with severe symptoms, but can also be short-lived and minimal.

Suggested Questions: Are there any parts of your body you would like me to avoid in this session? Are there any sensitives I should know?

Symptoms

- Patchy hair loss
- Could cause tingling or itching in affected areas before hair loss
- In some cases, nail changes

ANEMIA

Anemia is a condition characterized by a shortage of red blood cells, often due to deficiency of hemoglobin. Massage therapy is generally safe unless anemia is accompanied by other disorders that could be negatively affected by treatment.

PN- Clients with anemia may also face challenges such as nutritional deficiencies, increased inflammation in the body, & a higher susceptibility to infections.

Symptoms

- Fatigue
- Weakness
- Pale skin
- Shortness of breath
- Dizziness or lightheadedness
- Cold hands & feet
- Headaches
- Heart palpitations

Contraindications

- If accompanied with other disorders

ANKYLOSING SPONDYLITIS

This is a chronic inflammatory Arthritis (*see note* pg 22) that primarily affects the spine, however, it may affect other joints & organs.

PN-Avoid prolonged prone positioning if spinal stiffness is severe, and adjust bolstering as needed for comfort.

Suggested Questions: How are you managing symptoms? Are you seeing any chiropractic PCP or PT? What are your goals for massage therapy?Eg.Better ROM.

Symptoms

- Chronic back pain
- Limited ROM in Spine
- Joint pain
- Fatigue
- Enthesitis (Pain & inflammation where tendons & ligaments attach to bones)

Contraindications

- Stretching
- Cupping

AMPLIFIED MUSCULOSKELETAL PAIN SYNDROME (AMPS)

This is a condition where the nervous system overreacts to pain signals. This causes heightened pain perception & often spreads it throughout the body. AMPS is more common in children & adolescents, targeting 11-15 year olds.

PN- Because this pathology can't be seen, it is necessary to keep open communication in sessions.

Suggested Questions: How long have you been diagnosed? How are you managing your symptoms? Are you sensitive to heat or ice? What are your personal goals?

Symptoms

- Widespread Pain (can be 24hrs/7d/wk)
- Heightened sensitivity
- Fatigue
- Autonomic symptoms (swelling or color changes in the affected area, temperature differences in the skin, one area might feel colder or warmer)

ARTHRITIS

Arthritis is simply inflammation of the joints causing pain, stiffness and reduced mobility. The two most common types are: Osteoarthritis (OA) (see note pg 88): Wear-and-tear degeneration of cartilage & Rheumatoid Arthritis (RA)(see note pg 101): Autoimmune attack on joint linings.

PN-Arthritis is typically seen in older clients. Symptoms can flare, local contraindication rest of body can be massaged normally.

Suggested Questions: Are you taking any medications? What activities seem to make it worse?

Symptoms

- Joint pain
- Stiffness
- Swelling
- Reduced ROM

ANXIETY

This is a mental health condition characterized by constant feelings of worry, fear, or nervousness that can be situational, chronic, or related to a medical condition. Anxiety affects the nervous system and can manifest physically, emotionally, and behaviorally.

Suggested Questions: Does your client want to focus on reducing anxiety during the session? (would mean calmer slower motions & maybe aroma therapies)

Symptoms

- Increased heart rate (you can feel your heart beating "out of your chest")
- Muscle tension or aches
- Sweating or trembling
- Digestive issues, nausea, upset stomach
- Fatigue or difficulty sleeping (insomnia)

ASTHMA

Asthma is a chronic condition characterized by inflammation & narrowing of the airways. It can lead to difficulty breathing, wheezing, coughing, & shortness of breath. The severity of asthma attacks can vary: Mild cases may require an inhaler during strenuous activities like running, heavy workouts, or even laughing. Severe cases may require daily use of an inhaler for routine activities. Coughing tends to worsen during illness.

PN-Aromatherapy is generally not recommended for individuals with asthma, however, using a humidifier to add moisture to the air can help. Be cautious with positioning—some clients may feel discomfort lying prone for extended periods.

Suggested Questions: How long since you've been diagnosed? When do you find it brings the most difficulty? Do you have an inhaler on you?

Symptoms

- Shortness of breath (Dyspnea)
- Chest tightness
- Increased mucus production

Contraindications

- Aromatherapy
- Strongly scented emollients
- Prone position for an extended amount of time (varies)

ATHEROSCLEROSIS

Atherosclerosis is a condition in which plaque builds up in the arteries, leading to the narrowing and hardening of blood vessels. This is more common with age. DO NOT MASSAGE until cleared by PCP.

PN-It's best to avoid deep tissue work. Relaxation massage with lighter pressure is recommended.

Symptoms

- Chest pain
- Shortness of breath
- Weakness or numbness
- Stroke symptoms (make sure you know what a stroke looks like & call 911)
- Pain in the lower legs when walking

Contraindication

- Client should be cleared by PCP
- Deep tissue
- Gua sha
- Cupping

BAKER'S CYSTS

Baker's Cyst occurs when a synovial cyst (fluid-filled sac) in the popliteal fossa (back of the knee) becomes inflamed.

PN- The back of the knee is a local contraindication. Use caution, especially if there are signs of Thrombosis (see note pg 49), in which case a medical professional should be consulted.

Symptoms

- Visible Lump or swelling
- Pain
- Reduced range of motion

Contraindication Local

- Joint Mobilization/ stretching
- Deep tissue

BELL'S PALSY

This is a temporary weakness and/or paralysis of muscles on one side of the face due to inflammation of the facial nerve. This may look like a stroke and includes symptoms such as drooping of the mouth, inability to close the eye on affected side, inability to make full facial expressions. Bell's Palsy is normally caused by viral infections.

PN- If the client has been diagnosed with Bell's Palsy, it is not life threatening. If your client is showing similar symptoms, without a Bell's Palsy diagnosis, they may be having a stroke (call 911 immediately).

Symptoms

- Facial weakness or paralysis
- Pain around the jaw or behind the ear
- Tearing or drooping of the eyelid
- Sensory changes
- Difficulty smiling or frowning

Contraindications

- Face Massage
- Trigger Point work in neck

BONE SPURS

Also called Osteophytes, these bony growths develop along the edges of bones, typically in areas where bones meet other bones (i.e. joints). They are a common result of Osteoarthritis (see note pg 88) or other conditions that cause joint degeneration over time, although they can also form in other areas of the body.

PN- You will be able to see a bump, more common in feet due to gait or poor shoe choices. While the bone spurs themselves don't cause pain, rubbing against muscles will cause pain. Bone spurs have a risk of breaking off if enough force is put directly on them.

Suggested Questions: Do they give you pain? Have you seen a PCP about it & have they talked to you about any type of treatment to file it down?

Symptoms

- Pain
- Stiffness & limited mobility
- Swelling
- Decreased function in joint

Contraindications Local

- Deep Tissue

BUNIONS (HALLUX VALGUS)

A bunion is a bony bump that forms at the base of the big toe, often causing the toe to lean toward the second toe. This can lead to pain, swelling, & difficulty walking.

PN- Direct pressure on the bunion can cause pain & discomfort, especially if it's inflamed or irritated. Aggressive massage on the feet can potentially worsen pain, especially if the bunion is severe or inflamed.

Symptoms

- Visible Bump
- Swelling or Inflammation
- Calluses

Contraindication Local

- Deep Tissue
- Gua sha

BURSITIS

Bursitis just means (bursa inflammation.) Acute bursitis can be worse if intrusive specific massage irritates the area. This is a very common pathology, noted by different types.

Olecranon Bursitis (Elbow): Also known as "student's elbow", this is the swelling of the bursa over the elbow, often due to direct trauma or prolonged pressure.

Prepatellar Bursitis (Knee) nickname: Inflammation of the bursa in front of the kneecap, often caused by repetitive kneeling (e.g, construction work). nickname: water on knee.

Trochanteric Bursitis (Hip): Inflammation of the bursa on the outer side of the hip, often caused by excessive walking, running, or side-lying postures.

Retrocalcaneal Bursitis (Ankle): Inflammation of the bursa located between the calcaneus & achilles tendon, often due to repetitive stress or ill-fitting shoes.

Suggested Questions: Have you had any cortisone shots for this condition? How long have you been diagnosed? Does it bother you while doing a specific activity?

Symptoms for all
- Localized pain
- Swelling
- Warmth & redness (SHARP)
- Tenderness

Contraindications
- Local (while SHARP is present)

CANDIDIASIS

Candidiasis is a fungal infection that affects the skin, mucous membranes (nose, throat, mouth), and internal organs. There are different types when it affects different parts of the body. Oral (AKA Thrush), Cutaneous, Vaginal, Systemic. You can still have sessions with clients with Candidiasis; it's only local contraindication.

PN- It's also okay to reschedule the appointment until the virus has cleared, for precaution of other clients who are at higher risk of infection.

Suggested Question: Have you seen your PCP?

General symptoms: *VARYING*

- Irritation/inflammation
- Soreness
- Itchy
- Burning
- Fatigue

CARPAL TUNNEL SYNDROME

Entrapment of the median nerve between the carpal bones of the wrist & the transverse carpal ligament that holds down the flexor tendons. Pain in thumb, middle, and index finger. If massage can be conducted without risk of pain, then CTS is a local caution.

PN-Has the client been told about or has had the surgery. See neuromuscular therapist and/or collaborate with PT to better help clients needs.

Symptoms

- Numbness & tingling
- Pain/weakness
- "Shaking" of the hands (this is to try & get blood flow/tingling to stop in wrists)

Contraindications

- DT on joint
- Joint Mobilization
- Local if inflammation is active

CELLULITIS

This is a bacterial skin infection that affects the skin's deeper layers. Commonly occurs when bacteria enters the skin through a break or crack, such as a cut, surgical wound, or insect bite. Cellulitis can occur anywhere on the body, typically affecting the legs, face, and arms.

PN- This condition can't be passed by touch, however, it is still an active infection the client should wait until cleared by PCP.

Symptoms

- Redness & Swelling
- Pain or Tenderness
- Fever & Chills
- Blisters

Contraindications

- DO NOT MASSAGE

CERVICAL PALSY

This is a group of permanent neurological disorders caused by abnormal brain development or damage to the developing brain, affecting movement, muscle tone, & posture. While it is non-progressive (the brain injury does not worsen over time), the symptoms & secondary complications (like muscle contractures, joint deformities, or mobility issues) can change & require ongoing management.

Suggested Questions: Are you currently taking any medications? What would you like to get out of massage sessions? Are you working with a PT?

Symptoms

- Muscle stiffness/ Jerky movements
- Joint contractures (**local contraindication**)
- Poor coordination & Balance

CERVICAL RADICULOPATHY

This is a condition that occurs when a nerve in the cervical spine becomes compressed or irritated. It is commonly caused by Herniated Discs (see note pg 63), Bone Spurs, (see note pg 28) or other degenerative changes in the spine that press on the nerves as they exit the spinal column.

Symptoms
- Pain
- Numbness/tingling
- Weakness in the neck, shoulders, upper extremities

Contraindications
- Spine and neck work until cleared by PCP
- Stretching

CIRRHOSIS

A long term liver diease that occurs when the liver becomes heavily scarred. It is often caused by prolonged damage from alcohol use, Hepatitis,(see note pg 61) or fatty liver disease. As the liver becomes increasingly scarred, its ability to function properly declines, leading to complications such as jaundice (yellowing of the skin and whites of eyes), darkened urine, & pale-colored stool, ascites (fluid buildup in the abdomen), internal bleeding, & ultimately liver failure. Cirrhosis may affect liver enzyme levels, so any pressure applied to the abdomen or upper body could cause discomfort or exacerbation of liver function issues. DT or aggressive massage is not recommended on the abdomen.

PN- If fever or flu like symptoms are present, the client's session needs to be postponed.

Suggested Questions: Have you spoken to your PCP about massage? What are your goals with massage therapy?

Symptoms

- Edema (fluid retention)
- Flu-like symptoms (nausea &/or vomiting)
- Joint pain

Contraindications

- Abdominal work
- If flu like symptoms are present DO NOT MASSAGE

CHRONIC BRONCHITIS

This is a long-term inflammation of the bronchi that targets smokers & attacks the lungs.

DO NOT MASSAGE clients until they have been cleared by PCP

Symptoms

- Persistent cough
- Mucus production
- Chest tightness
- Cyanosis *(in advanced stages)* (A bluish/grey color around the lips or fingertips, indicating low oxygen levels in the blood.)

Contraindications

- DO NOT MASSAGE

CHRONIC PELVIC PAIN SYNDROME

This is persistent or recurrent pain in the pelvic region lasting six months or longer, affecting both men & women. There are many causes for this condition, ranging from reproductive & urinary issues to gastrointestinal & musculoskeletal problems. The pain may be constant or intermittent.

Suggested Questions: Are you taking any medication to help with this condition? Would you want to do any focus work including stretching the muscles that support the pelvis? Does heat help pain?

Symptoms

- Persistent or intermittent pain
- Pain with intercourse
- Pelvic pressure or heaviness
- Urinary symptoms

Contraindications

- Abdominal work

COMPARTMENT DISORDER

Acute Compartment Syndrome occurs when an injury or repetitive stress causes a dangerous increase in pressure within a muscle compartment. These compartments contain muscles, nerves & blood vessels enclosed by a tough layer of fascia. This pressure can damage or destroy muscle & nerve cells. It is a serious condition that needs quick medical care. Clients with symptoms like severe pain (worse than expected), numbness, tingling, difficulty moving, swelling, or pale, tight skin should be referred out immediately.

*PN-*The chances of this occurring during a session are extremely low. This is included so that if a client mentions having had it, you understand their experience.

Symptoms

- Severe, unrelenting pain
- Swelling
- Paleness or coolness
- Numbness or tingling (Paresthesia)
- Shiny, tight skin

Contraindication

- **MEDICAL EMERGENCY**

COMPLEX REGIONAL PAIN SYNDROME(CRPS)

Previously known as Reflex Sympathetic Dystrophy (RSD), is a chronic pain condition that typically affects a limb after an injury, though it can also occur without an obvious injury. It is characterized by severe pain that is out of proportion to the original injury or trauma, along with a variety of sensory, motor, & autonomic symptoms.

Suggested Questions: Have you had a massage before? Has pressure been a challenge for you? Have you been cleared by a PCP?

CRPS-I (formerly RSD):

- This type occurs after an injury where no nerve damage is evident

CRPS-II (formerly Causalgia):

- This type occurs after an injury where there is evident nerve damage

Symptoms

- Swelling
- Skin changes
- Sensitive to Pain/Pressure

Contraindications

- Local until cleared by PCP

(COPD)EMPHYSEMA

A chronic lung condition that causes shortness of breath. After a long period, this condition can damage the thin walls of the air sacs in the lungs. It is most commonly caused by smoking or long-term exposure to air pollutants. This is a group of diseases known as chronic obstructive pulmonary disease (COPD). This condition results in a loss of lung elasticity, making it harder for the lungs to expand & contract efficiently, which limits airflow & oxygen intake.

PN- Think of asthma but more extreme. Emphysema can lead to respiratory failure and can cause death if untreated. DO NOT MASSAGE clients until they have been cleared by PCP

Symptoms

- Shortness of Breath (Dyspnea)
- Chest Tightness
- Barrel Chest(barrel like shaped chest)
- Cyanosis is a bluish/grey color around the lips or fingertips,(low oxygen levels in the blood.)

Contraindication

- DO NOT MASSAGE until cleared by PCP

CROHN'S DISEASE

Crohn's Disease is a bowel disease that causes chronic inflammation of the digestive tract. The inflammation can affect any part of the gastrointestinal tract, from the mouth to the anus. The most common is ileocolitis which targets the large intestine.

PN-Clients with Crohn's Disease are most likely to be dehydrated from this since they arent able to absorb fluids like normal. A general rule of thumb for water intake is multiply body weight by .5 to get an estimate of many ounces you should have in a day. Half your body weight in ounces.

Suggested Questions: What is your daily water intake? When are your symptoms worse?

Symptoms

- Abdominal pain
- Weight loss
- Fatigue
- Malnutrition
- Changes in stool color/diarrhea

Contraindication

- Abdominal work

DIABETES MELLITUS

This is a chronic condition where the body either doesn't produce enough insulin (Type 1), or can't use insulin effectively (Type 2).

PN- Avoid deep tissue massage over insulin injection sites. Be cautious of sensory impairments in extremities to prevent injury.

Suggested Questions: How long have you been diagnosed with diabetes? Have you ever been hosptalized with serious symptoms? How do you normally track your numbers? Are you seeing a diabetic coach? Where is your injection site? (typically the abdomen)

Symptoms:

- Fatigue
- Frequent urination
- Excessive thirst
- Slow wound healing

DISC DISEASE

The nucleus pulposus (center of the spine) & or other parts of the disc extends beyond its normal borders.

PN- Disc problems can be complex & difficult to pin down; these are situations where massage therapists can benefit most by working as part of a healthcare team.

Symptoms

- Local back pain
- Radiating pain (*Sciatica*) (see note pg 103)
- Numbness/tingling

Contraindications

- Work on spine
- Stretching

DUPUYTREN'S CONTRACTURE (PALMAR FIBROMATOSIS)

Dupuytren's contracture, also known as Palmar fibromatosis or Viking's disease, is a condition where the connective tissue thickens and tightens over time, making it hard to straighten the fingers. Making it hard to move the fingers. If nerves are damaged, feeling in the hand could be reduced, which means massage is a caution.

PN-If client has a lack of feeling in hand, caution & extra communication need to be present.

Suggested Questions:When were you diagnosed? What are your goals for massage therapy?Are you taking any medications for the condition?

Symptoms

- Small, firm lumps or nodules in the palm *(Palmar Nodules)*
- Thickened Palmar Fascia
- Decreased hand function

DIVERTICULAR DISEASE

This is the presence of small pouches (diverticula) that form in the walls of the colon. Most individuals with Diverticula don't experience symptoms. However, if the pouches become inflamed or infected, it can lead to a condition called Diverticulitis. If an individual has an active infection or inflammation in the diverticula (colon), massage can increase pain and should be avoided. Abdominal massage might trigger nausea or digestive discomfort, particularly if the person is experiencing a flare-up.

PN- Always check in with their PCP to better plan their sessions with their needs/goals.

Symptoms

- Abdominal pain
- Fever
- Digestive disturbances

Contraindications

- Abdominal work
- If flu-like symptoms are present DO NOT MASSAGE

DYSTONIA

This is a common condition that involves repetitive involuntary- sometimes sustained-muscle tightening. Sudden twitching, jerking, or twisting movements during the session. Uncontrollable postures or muscle contractions that may shift positioning. Repetitive movements that may make it difficult for them to stay still. 250,000 Americans are diagnosed every year making it the third most common movement disorder in the U.S. Dystonia can affect a single muscle, a group of muscles, or all of the muscles in the body.

PN- If a client frequently moves or twist, be prepared to adjust your approach and positioning throughout the session.

Symptoms

- Twisting & repetitive movements
- Tremors
- Voice problems
- A dragging foot
- Pain

ECZEMA

Skin condition, often appearing as dry, inflamed, blistered, crusted, or scaly (flaky skin), often presenting as a combination of these symptoms. Eczema may affect localized areas or spread across the entire body. In some cases, Gua sha can lead to the skin weeping clear fluid. There are multiple types of this condition, confirm diagnosis & of which type of Eczema. If the flare-up is localized to one area, the client is still able to receive massage on unaffected parts of the body.

PN- Clients may be hypersensitive to scented lotions & oils. All allergies, irritants, drastic weather, stress, & being sick can all trigger symptoms.

Symptoms

- Itchy skin (Pruritus)
- Red, inflamed skin
- Dry, flaky skin
- Weeping or oozing skin

Contraindication

- Local

EMBOLISM (PE) & THROMBOSIS (DVT)

An embolism is a traveling clot or group of debris. Thrombosis is a blood clot inside the blood vessel restricting blood flow. Embolism and Thrombosis are connected. A person with thrombosis is at risk of developing an embolism if the clot dislodges. Not all thromboses leads to embolisms, and embolisms can come from other sources (like air, fat, or amniotic fluid). If a client has a history of deep vein thrombosis (DVT), they may be at risk for pulmonary embolism (PE), which is a serious complication.

PN- Clients may be taking blood thinners, they also carry more risk with bruising. If unsure where they have blood clots DO NOT MASSAGE.

Suggested Questions: Are you currently in treatment? When was last treatment? What symptoms are affecting you most? What are your goals in massage? Have you been cleared by a PCP?

Symptoms
- Swelling in the affected area
- Red or discolored skin
- Engorged veins
- Rapid heart rate *(Tachycardia)*
- Sudden numbness/& or weakness
- Loss of vision

Contraindication
- If not being treated DO NOT MASSAGE

ENCEPHALITIS (WEST NILE VIRUS)

Inflammation of the brain, often due to infection (herpes simplex). The client may have zero symptoms or flu-like symptoms. Be aware clients may have muscle weakness, problems with coordination, be disoriented, & may have nausea. This condition needs immediate medical attention. Client needs to be cleared by PCP before massage session.

Suggested Questions: How long were you hospitalized? Do you have any lasting symptoms that bring challenges now? Memory concerns, weakneakness, or numbness?

Symptoms

- Severe headache
- Confusion or disorientation
- Seizures
- Sensitivity to light *(Photophobia)*

Contraindication

- DO NOT MASSAGE until cleared by PCP

EHLERS-DANLOS SYNDROME

A group of genetic disorders affecting connective tissues, leading to joint hypermobility, skin fragility, & potential vascular complications. These clients are prone to dislocation of joints.

PN- Ehlers-Danlos syndrome is an umbrella term for wide range of hypermobility conditions. Your client does not need to be stretched they are hypermobile they will just keep going. In rare cases clients with Ehlers-Danlos Syndrome (EDS) may have vascular EDS (vEDS), a genetic connective tissue disorder that makes blood vessels and organs fragile and more prone to injury.

Symptoms

- Stretchy skin (in some types).
- Fragile blood vessels are prone to rupture *(vEDS)*
- Hypermobility

Contraindications

- Joint mobilization
- Stretching

ENDOMETRIOSIS

Endometriosis is a condition where tissue similar to the lining of the uterus (endometrium) grows outside the uterus, typically in the pelvic cavity. These growths can spread to other areas, including the abdomen, & in rare cases, even above the diaphragm. May cause scarring & adhesions in the pelvic cavity.

PN-Therapists should take special caution & care when doing anything more than superficial work on the abdomen.

Symptoms
- Painful periods
- Pain during intercourse *(Dyspareunia)*
- Pain with bowel movements/urination
- Fatigue, nausea, or diarrhea

Contraindication
- Abdominal work

FIBROID TUMORS

Fibroid tumors, or (leiomyomas), are non-cancerous growths that develop in or on the uterus. They can vary in size & may cause symptoms such as, heavy menstrual bleeding, pelvic pain, & pressure on surrounding organs. Direct or deep pressure on the abdomen can exacerbate pain or discomfort, especially if fibroids are large or inflamed.

Suggested Questions: Are you scheduled for surgery? Are you currently taking any medications? Have you been cleared by a PCP for massage?

Symptoms

- Painful periods *(Dysmenorrhea)*
- Frequent urination
- Constipation

Contraindication

- Abdomin work

FIBROMYALGIA

Describes a complex condition involving problems with neurotransmitters, hormone imbalances, sleep disorders. Pain can be felt in muscles, tendons, ligaments, & other soft tissues. Chronic widespread & unpredictable pain.

PN- Every client with fibromyalgia is different, some may want Swedish pressure, others may need more pressure to feel relief. Remember, people with chronic pain have a different pain scale. Keep open communication throughout session. Try broader tools such as forearms, full palms, & Gua sha. Dispersing pressure to avoid a fibro attack.

Symptoms

- Widespread pain
- Cognitive difficulties *("Fibro Fog")*
- Tender points

GALLSTONES

Gallstones are solid particles that form in the gallbladder and can vary in size. They are made of cholesterol or bile fragments. Some people with gallstones don't experience any symptoms *(asymptomatic)*. Abdominal massage can also trigger nausea or digestive distress. In rare cases, deep pressure in the abdominal area may increase the risk of complications, such as a gallstone attack or biliary colic. Biliary Colic refers to severe pain caused by a gallstone blocking the bile duct, leading to spasms or blockage in the gallbladder clients may complain of sharp pain in the upper abdomen, nausea, and vomiting.

PN- If client is in extreme pain move session until cleared by PCP.

Symptoms

- Pain
- Nausea
- Inflammation if the stones block bile ducts

Contraindication

- Abdominal work

GANGLION CYSTS

Small connective tissue pouches filled with fluid that develope on joint capsules or tendinous sheaths. Massage is a local contraindication.

PN- This is also called "bible cysts" some clients may want ti hit it with a book to get rid of it. This is not recommended and could cause more harm to other structures.

Symptoms
- Visible lump
- Pain
- Numbness/ tingling
- Reduced ROM

Contraindication
- Local

GASTROENTERITIS

Inflammation of the stomach & intestines, typically caused by viral or bacterial infections, often referred to as stomach flu. It is typically transmitted through contaminated food, water, or contact with infected individuals. Postpone session with client with active infection.

Symptoms

- Nausea & vomiting
- Headache
- Dehydration
- Abdominal cramps

Contraindication

- DO NOT MASSAGE until cleared by PCP

GOUT

Joint inflammation related to chemical imbalances. If a client complains of pain & shows extreme inflammation around a joint, consult a PCP before applying ice, which will promote crystallization if it's gout. No bodywork that involves manipulation, traction, & pressure on a infected joint may make the situation worse.

PN- Gout is in the same family as arthritis (see note pg 22).

Symptoms

- Joint pain
- Inflammation
- Stiff joints
- Limited ROM

GRAVES DISEASE

Graves' disease is an autoimmune disorder that causes the thyroid gland to overproduce hormones (hyperthyroidism). This can affect metabolism, energy levels, & overall health.

PN- The neck/throat on these clients may be swollen due to the thyroid glands being the main problem area with this pathology. Neck work is contraindicated.

Symptoms

- Increased heart rate (tachycardia)
- Tremors in hands or fingers
- Heat intolerance & excessive sweating
- Weight loss despite normal or increased appetite
- Bulging eyes (exophthalmos) in some cases
- Fatigue & muscle weakness

Contraindication

- Anterior neck work

HAMMERTOE

Foot deformity that affects the second, third & fourth toes. If a client's foot is hot, painful & inflamed, this is a local contraindication for any work. Does not affect the rest of the body unless other pathology is also noted.

Symptoms
- Swelling & Redness
- Reduced ROM

Contraindication
- Local if SHARP is present

HEPATITIS (A, B & C)

This is inflammation of the liver, often caused by a viral infection, but it can also result from alcohol use, toxins, medications, or autoimmune conditions. Common types include Hepatitis A, B, & C.

- HAV- Consuming contaminated food or water, It travels from person to person only from the fecal-oral route; & isn't typically chronic. This is a very low risk of transmission in massage settings.
- (HBV)- Is a viral infection, can be transmitted by blood, semen, or other bodily fluids. Use universal precautions if the client has open wounds or blood exposure.
- HCV- Viral infection, often chronic, only passed by blood-to-blood contact. Use regular precautions; the risk of transmission in massage settings is low with proper hygiene practices.

Symptoms for all
- Fatigue
- Jaundice (yellowing of the skin & eyes)
- Nausea, vomiting, or abdominal pain
- Dark urine, pale stools
- Joint pain (in some cases)

HERNIA

Hernia translates to "protrusion". There are a variety of hernias that can occur in the body. Local contraindication for massage. Since the wall is already compromised & extra pressure or stretching may make this worse. Common hernia placements include,(inguinal:groin, hiatal:stomach & inclucional: from surgery)

PN-See ANMT therapist for recommendations for collaboration.

Suggested Questions: When were you diagnosed? Was it due to an accident? Have you been cleared by a PCP for massage?

Symptoms

- Visible Bulge
- Weakness or Pressure
- Redness or Tenderness

Contraindication

- Local

HERNIATED DISC

A condition where the soft inner portion of an intervertebral disk (nucleus pulposus) bulges or ruptures through the outer layer, pressing on nearby nerves. This can be caused by injury, osteoporosis, (see note pg 87) or poor posture (either overuse or incorrect alignment).

Symptoms

- Local or radiating pain (commonly in the neck, lower back, or legs)
- Numbness, tingling, or weakness in affected areas

HIV/AIDS

(Human Immunodeficiency Virus) attacks the immune system, weakening the body's ability to fight infections. If left untreated, it can develop into AIDS (Acquired Immunodeficiency Syndrome), where the immune system becomes severely compromised, at a higher risk of infection. People with HIV/AIDS may experience skin sensitivity or rashes, aggressive DT may irritate the skin.

PN- other than the client being at an increased risk for getting sick there are no other contraindications. If they have other pathologies that need attention or caution with the session, look at other notes.

Symptoms
- Flu-like symptoms
- Headache
- Gastrointestinal problems
- Sore throat & mouth sores

HIVES

These are raised, red or skin-colored welts that appear on the skin, often accompanied by itching. Usually triggered by an allergic reaction or other factors that cause histamine and related chemicals to be released into the skin. Hives can range in size, last for hours to days, & may come & go. DO NOT MASSAGE clients with hives. Can cause it to become worse, with lotions & skin irritation.

Symptoms
- Welts
- Itching
- Swelling

Contraindication
- DO NOT MASSAGE until hives are gone

HYPERKYPHOSIS

This is an exaggerated forward curvature of the thoracic (upper) spine, resulting in a rounded or hunched back appearance. While a certain degree of kyphosis is normal, hyperkyphosis is when the curve exceeds 50 degrees.

Suggested Questions: Are you currently in treatment for this condition?

PN-opposite to Hypokyphosis(see note pg 68)

Symptoms

- Postural changes
- Back pain
- Breathing problems

HYPERTENSION

Known as high blood pressure, chronic condition where blood pushes too hard against the walls of the arteries. Over time, this can damage blood vessels, the heart, kidneys, & brain. Increasing the risk of cardiovascular diseases, stroke, kidney disease, & other complications.

PN- This is specifically if it's untreated. Not if it is being treated/managed.

Symptoms

- Headaches
- Dizziness or lightheadedness
- Blurred or double vision
- Shortness of breath
- Nosebleeds
- Chest pain
- Fatigue
- Heart palpitations

HYPOKYPHOSIS

Refers to a reduced or flattened natural curvature of the thoracic spine, leading to a abnormal spinal shape.The spine has an exaggerated forward curvature (flatback appearance).

PN- opposite to Hyperkyphosis(see note pg 66)

Symptoms

- Postural changes
- Back pain
- Breathing problems
- Neck strain or headache

HYPOTHYROIDISM

A condition in which the thyroid gland produces insufficient amounts of thyroid hormones, leading to a slowed metabolism & a range of bodily dysfunctions.

PN- Women on hormonal treatment (HRT) for menopause (see note pg 127) may have a higher risk of developing hypothyroidism.

Symptoms

- Fatigue
- Weight gain
- Cold intolerance
- Hair loss

INFLUENZA

Is a contagious viral infection that affects the respiratory system, causing symptoms like fever, chills, body aches, sore throat, cough, & fatigue. DO NOT MASSAGE clients until they have been cleared by PCP

Symptoms
- Fever/Chills
- Sweating
- Cough
- Headache
- Shortness of breath

Contraindication
- DO NOT MASSAGE

IRRITABLE BOWEL SYNDROME(IBS)

A chronic gastrointestinal disorder that affects the large intestine. It is characterized by symptoms such as abdominal pain, bloating, gas, & changes in bowel habits, including diarrhea, constipation, or alternating between both. Abdominal massage or intense pressure can sometimes cause discomfort, particularly during active flare-ups when the intestines are sensitive.

PN- Abdominal massage is typically a local contraindication during a flare. If your client isn't in a flare light abdominal massage has the same benefits as anyone else.

Symptoms

- Bloating & gas
- Diarrhea
- Constipation
- Fatigue & difficulty sleeping

Contraindication

- Abdominal work

JOINT REPLACEMENT SURGERY

Arthroplasty is a procedure to repair articulating surfaces within a synovial joint. New joint replacements carry specific risks in relation to surgical complications, infection, blood clots & incomplete healing. Older replacements must be carefully maneuvered to avoid stressing joints.

PN- Joint replacements typically have a lifespan of 7-10 years. Ask your client if their PCP has discussed the possibility of future surgery.

Symptoms

- Swelling
- Grinding sensation *(Crepitus)*
- Poor response to non-surgical treatments

Contraindications

- Stretching the joint
- Deep Tissue on joint

KELOID SCARS

A type of raised, thick, & fibrous scar that forms as a result of overactive wound healing. They occur when the skin produces excessive collagen during the healing process, leading to a growth that extends beyond the original wound boundaries.

PN- Keloid scars don't typically hurt the client unless they grow too large to get caught on clothes. Non-contagious

Symptoms

- Raised, thickened scar
- Shiny or smooth appearance
- Itching or tenderness
- Dark pigmentation

KIDNEY STONES

Also called *(Renal Calculi)*, these solid, crystalline mineral deposits form in the kidneys. They can vary in size & may cause severe pain when they move through the urinary tract. Kidney stones can lead to obstruction of the urinary tract, causing pain & other complications if not treated. DO NOT MASSAGE ABDOMEN until stones have passed & the client is cleared by PCP.

PN- Kidney stones typically can be passed without intervention from PCP, however, some stones that are too large may need to be broken up by PCP.

Symptoms

- Severe, sharp pain
- Blood in urine
- Frequent urination or urgency

Contraindication

- Abdominal work

KIDNEY DISEASE (POLYCYSTIC KIDNEY DISEASE, PYELONEPHRITIS, & RENAL FAILURE)

A condition in which the kidneys are damaged & cannot function effectively. Kidney diseases are categorized based on their progression, underlying causes, & the rate at which kidney function declines.

PN- Lighter massage is recommended. Deep tissue on the lower back may cause more kidney sensitivity.

Symptoms

- Decreased urine output
- Swelling in legs, ankles, or feet.
- Fatigue
- Confusion

Contraindications

- Abdominal work
- Deep Tissue on lower back

LUPUS

An autoimmune disease where the body's immune system mistakenly attacks healthy tissue, causing widespread inflammation. It can affect various organs including the skin, joints, kidneys, heart, & lungs.

PN- Clients might have more sensitivity to touch, & experience fatigue & inflammation flare-ups. Most clients experience body aches making their muscles tender; in turn making firm pressure uncomfortable. Keep open communication during the entire session. Heat therapy may help with some symptoms/pain. Lymphatic work, can be beneficial to these clients as well.

Symptoms

- Joint pain/tenderness
- Photosensitivity (sensitive to sunlight causing rashes)
- Hair loss
- Kidney, heart & respiratory issues
- General discomfort

LYME DISEASE

Infection caused by a spirochete bacterium called Borrelia Burgdorferi. Commonly affected by a (tick bite) The arthritic phase involves intermittently severe, painful inflammation of joints, this contraindicates massage. Can also affect the cardiovascular (heart) system potentially causing heart palpitations or irregular heart rhythms (known as Lyme carditis), which is a serious complication.

PN- Clients with chronic lyme disease can receive massage. It should be noted that these clients may have pressure sensitivity.

Symptoms

- Early sign-bull's-eye-shaped rash
- Flu-like symptoms
- Neurological(Facial palsy *(Bell's Palsy)*)Numbness, tingling, or shooting pain in limbs
- Late symptoms Severe Joint Pain & Swelling
- Persistent fatigue/Difficulty sleeping

Contraindication

- DO NOT MASSAGE until cleared by PCP

LYMPHEDEMA

Lymphedema is a chronic medical condition characterized by swelling (edema) that occurs when the lymphatic system is impaired & unable to properly drain lymph fluid. If there is an active infection DO NOT MASSAGE until they're cleared by PCP.

PN- If client is cleared by PCP no infection is present lighter massage distal to affected area is recommended.

Symptoms

- Swelling
- Skin changes
- Frequent infections

Contraindication

- DO NOT MASSAGE if client has an active infection

LYMPHANGITIS

An infection with inflammation in the lymphangitis (segments of the lymphatic vessel between two valves) DO NOT MASSAGE clients until they have been cleared by physician. Clients will have fever, general malaise throbbing pain, & edema at the site of infection.

PN- Clients in recovery can receive massage.

Symptoms

- Red streaks on the skin
- Pain & tenderness
- Fever & chills
- Enlarged lymph nodes

Contraindication

- DO NOT MASSAGE until cleared by PCP

METATARSALGIA

Metatarsalgia is a painful condition affecting the ball of the foot. It occurs when the nerves becomes inflamed & irritated by pressure against the metatarsal bones. Commonly seen in clients who wear uncomfortable shoes. (ie.)High heels, work boots, ballet slippers, rock climber shoes.

PN- The feet can be massaged, just keep open communication on pressure.

Symptoms

- Pain in the ball of the foot, often flared when walking or standing
- Tenderness & swelling
- Numbness or tingling in the toe

MIGRAINE DISORDER

A neurological condition that causes moderate to severe headaches, often accompanied by additional symptoms. Migraines can last from hours to days & may significantly impact daily life.

PN- Some clients may tell you they know a migraine is coming, others may have more spontaneous episodes.

Suggested Questions: How often are your headaches? Do you have specific triggers? Do you know when they start to come on? Is there anything you've done that makes them better? Anything that doesn't help? Have you been diagnosed with chronic migraines or do you get them every once in a while?

Symptoms
- Throbbing or pulsing pain, often on one side of the head
- Aura (sensory disubances)
- Nausea or vomiting
- Sensitivity to light, sound, or smell
- Fatigue & mood changes (before or after an attack)

MONONUCLEOSIS

Also known as (Mono) this is a viral infection that begins in the salivary glands & throat & then moves into the lymphatic system. DO NOT MASSAGE until they have been cleared by PCP.

PN- After the client has been cleared lighter massage is recommended.

Symptoms

- Fever
- Inflamed lymph nodes
- General malaise (not feeling like themselves, unwell)

Contraindication

- DO NOT MASSAGE until cleared by PCP

MORTON'S NEUROMA

This is when the connective tissue sheath that encases the common digital nerves of the toes thickens. "Nerve tumor". Squeezing the metatarsal heads may elicit symptoms.

PN- With this pathology, the rest of the body can be treated like normal if there are no other pathologies that say otherwise.

Suggested Questions: What shoes do they wear? Are you always moving for work or are you at a desk?

Symptoms

- Pain in the ball of the foot
- Tingling/numbness
- Feeling of a lump or pebble while walking
- Swelling

Contraindications

- Deep Tissue on feet
- Gua sha on affected foot

MULTIPLE SCLEROSIS

MS is a chronic autoimmune disease that affects the central nervous system. It causes the immune system to attack the protective covering of nerve fibers leading to communication issues between the brain & the body.

PN- MS is a progressive disease, be kind to those clients with this (as you would anyone else) also make sure open communication about positioning & pressure throughout the entire session.

Symptoms

- Muscle weakness
- Vision problems
- Coordination/mobility issues
- Fatigue
- Prone to being hot

MUSCULAR DYSTROPHY

Muscular Dystrophy (MD) is a group of several closely related neuromuscular diseases caused by genetic mutations that result in the progressive degeneration of muscle tissue. Clients may generally be frail with a risk of osteoporosis depending on their age. Advanced cases with serious symptoms may involve heart & respiratory weakness.

Suggested Questions: Any medications for pain management? What do they want out of massage therapy? Has your PCP done any imaging tests? Are you in PT for the meantime.

Symptoms

- Muscle weakness
- Waddling gait
- Difficulty standing or rising
- Enlarged calves (*Pseudohypertrophy*)
- Joint contractures

Contraindications

- Deep Tissue
- Gua sha
- Cupping

OSGOOD-SCHLATTER DISEASE

This condition happens when the quadriceps tendon attaches to the shin bone (tibia) & becomes irritated or inflamed. This is a very common condition in children & teens, especially those who are very active. The client may say it's worse when being active,(running, jumping, or kneeling.)

PN- Adults don't have this condition however, they can have lingering effects from this condition such as a bony bump on the tibia that causes discomfort & in rare cases chronic pain or sensitivity in the area especially after being active or kneeling.

Symptoms

- Pain
- Swelling
- Tender to the touch

OSTEOPOROSIS (POROUS BONES)

"Porous Bones" Calcium is pulled off the bones faster than replaced leaving them thin, brittle & prone to injury. Often called a "silent disease" because it may not show symptoms until a fracture occurs. Primary risk fracture of bones. Other pathologies may apply. It is most common in older adults, particularly women after menopause, though men can also develop the condition. Common areas affect the spine, hips & wrists.

Symptoms

- Bone fractures, normally in joints
- Chronic back pain
- Height loss
- Stooped Posture

Contraindications

- Stretching
- Deep Tissue

OSTEOARTHRITIS

This Is the most common form of arthritis. Loss of cartilage in synovial joints. Acute inflammation contraindicates massage that may exacerbate symptoms but this is rare.

PN- This is a local contradindication.

Symptoms

- Joint pain
- Stiffness
- Swelling
- Decreased ROM in affected joints

Contraindications local

- Stretching
- Deep Tissue on bones

PERIPHERAL NEUROPATHY

Peripheral nerves, either singly or in groups, are damaged or irritated through lack of blood circulation, chemical imbalance & other factors. If the client is complaining of pain, tingling, or numbness they should be cleared by a PCP for massage. Numbness can reduce the sensation of feeling in the body & therefore clients can not give an accurate depiction of pressure.

Causes of this pathology are as follows: Diabetes(see note pg 43): (this is the most common), trauma or compression of nerves (e.g. carpal tunnel syndrome)(see note pg 32); Shingles (Zoster)(see note pg 124), Lyme disease(see note pg 77), HIV.(see note pg 64) Chemotherapy, alcohol, and heavy metals. Autoimmune diseases (e.g.,lupus), vitamin deficiencies, or Kidney Disease, (see note pg 75) are also known causes.

Symptoms

- Numbness or tingling ("pins & needles")
- Heightened sensitivity to touch (*allodynia*)
- Loss of sensation, especially in the extremities
- Weakness or loss of muscle control
- Difficulty walking or coordinating movements
- Severe sweating, blood pressure, or digestion (in some cases)

Contraindications

- Deep Tissue
- Gua sha
- Cupping

PEPTIC ULCER

A Peptic ulcer is an open sore that develops on the lining of the stomach, small intestine, or esophagus. Intense pressure on the abdominal area may cause nausea or vomiting in some individuals, particularly if the ulcer is active or causing pain. Stay away from abdomen work unless cleared by PCP.

PN- Blood clots (see note pg 49) are always a local contraindication.

Suggested Questions: Do you currently have blood clots, where?.

Symptoms

- Sesceptible bruising & bleeding
- Itchy Skin *(Pruritus)*
- Loss of Appetite & Weight Loss
- Confusion or Memory Problems (Hepatic Encephalopathy)
- Jaundice

Contraindications

- Abdomen
- Where blood clots are present local

PES PLANUS, PES CAVUS (FLAT & HIGH ARCH FOOT)

Meaning "flat feet". Lack of medial arch between the calcaneus & the great toe. These clients are often connected to an underlying disorder that might require special attention.

PN-Podiatry may need to be part of the plan for your. Also keep in mind if there is no support in one of both feet how that may affect the rest of the body in gait (walking), knees, & hips. When uncertain referout.

Symptoms

- Tired/aching feet
- Discomfort in most shoes
- Shin splints (see note pg 107)
- Leg, knee, & lower back pain (think of the kinetic chain)

PLANTAR FASCIITIS

Keep in mind that 1-10 people at some point in their lives will have this diagnosis. Inflammation of the bottom of the foot muscles. Clients may experience stabbing pain in the heel or arch of the foot, & swelling on the bottom of the heel. Can be an acute or chronic condition. If a client uses cortisone injections to treat the site, massage is contraindicated until tissues have stabilized.

PN- The client is likely to be stuck in dorsiflexion or plantar flexion;make note of ROM. This doesn't mean that every client that is stuck in plantar or dorsiflexion has plantar fasciitis. I wanted to note how common this is due to wearing heels, runners, & people who don't have proper foot support with high arches.

Symptoms

- Foot pain more targeted in the heel or arch of the foot
- Increased pain after exercise
- Swelling

Contraindication

- Local (if SHARP is present)

PNEUMONIA

A lung infection that causes inflammaation and fluid build up in the air sacs *(alveoli)* in one or both lungs, This can cause coughing, difficulty breathing & chest pain. DO NOT MASSAGE clients until they have been cleared by PCP.

Symptoms

- Cough
- Fever/chills
- Difficulty breathing

Contraindication

- DO NOT MASSAGE until cleared by PCP

POLYCYSTIC KIDNEY DISEASE

(PKD) is a genetic disorder characterized by the growth of numerous cysts in the kidneys. These fluid-filled cysts can vary in size & may impair kidney function over time. PKD is one of the most common inherited kidney diseases, leading to chronic Kidney Disease (see note pg 75) or kidney failure in many individuals.

Symptoms

- Abdominal pain
- High blood pressure
- Kidney stones (see note pg 74)

Contraindication

- Abdominal work

POSTURAL ORTHOSTATIC TACHYCARDIA SYNDROME (POTS)

POTS, is a condition in which the autonomic nervous system is dysregulated. Be aware that prolonged supine positions lying flat can reduce blood flow to the brain causing a flare-up in symptoms. Side-lying or seated massage may be more comfortable.

PN- Be mindful shorter sessions are encouraged. Encourage rest after the session so the client can obtain massage work & not exacerbate symptoms. Hot stones & heat therapies aren't recommended due to the clients nervous system already being overworked.

Symptoms

- Increased heart rate
- Dizziness & lightheadedness
- Fatigue/nausea
- Fainting or near-fainting
- Brain Fog/headache
- Muscle weakness
- Can also feel extremely hot or cold

Contraindication

- Hot stones/ Heat therapy

PROSTATITIS

Inflammation of the prostate gland. It can be acute or chronic & is often caused by bacterial infection, rarely nonbacterial. If the client has an active infectio, they need to be cleared by a PCP & postponed session until infection has passed.

Symptoms

- Flu-like symptoms in acute cases
- Pain with intercourse
- General pain in lower back, pelvic area, or genitals

Contraindication

- IF infection is present DONT MASSAGE

PSORIASIS

Psoriasis is a chronic autoimmune condition that causes skin cells to multiply too quickly, leading to thick, scaly patches on the skin. It can appear anywhere on the body, however, is often found on the scalp, elbows, & knees. Is associated with redness, itching, & inflammation.

Suggested Questions: Are there any emollients that you're sensitive to? Are you okay with hot towels?

Symptoms

- Redness/Inflammation
- Itching
- Overheating/sweating

Contraindications

- Gua sha
- Cupping

PTSD (POST TRAMATIC STRESS DISORDER)

PTSD is a mental health conditon triggerd by expirencing or witnessing a traumatic event. It can cause intense emotional & physical reactions that persist long after the event. During an episode, a client may relive the trauma, expirencing flashbacks dissociation, or loss of emotional and physical control. *PN-* You do not need to ask if they are seeing a psychologist, now if the client brings up, suicidal thoughts, or thoughts of harming themselves or others use your voice to tell a mental specialist. (this goes with any time a client brings this up)

RAYNAUD'S DISEASE

Is a vascular disorder causing temporary narrowing of blood vessels, primarily in fingers & toes, in response to cold or stress. It can be primary (idiopathic) or secondary (associated with other conditions like autoimmune diseases).

Suggested Questions: Would you like an extra blanket or higher table warmer setting? Do you have any sensitivity, lack of sensitivity in your hands & feet right now?

Symptoms

- Skin color changes(blue,purple,white)
- Numbness tingling
- Sensitivity to cold

RAYNAUD'S PHENOMENON

Raynaud's phenomenon is very similar to Raynaud's Disease (see note pg 99), but it carries more risks & complications and typically affects adults 30 years or older. This is tied to autoimmune disorders that affects the fingers and toes. During an episode blood vessels narrow for an extended period of time which can lead to skin and soft tissue damage.

PN- Clients with this have a higher chance of getting ulcers especially in sever cases.

Suggested Questions: Would you like an extra blanket or higher table warmer setting? Do you have any sensitivity, lack of sensitivity in your hands & feet right now? Has a PCP talked about any ulcers in your body?

Symptoms

- Triggered by cold or stress
- Tingling or pain
- Skin color changes(blue,purple white)

RHEUMATOID ARTHRITIS

Chronic autoimmune disease is where the body's immune system attacks healthy joints, causing inflammation, pain, stiffness, & eventually joint damage. It typically affects joints in the hands, wrists, knees, & feet, & can lead to deformities & reduced range of motion over time. The client may have had a joint replacement surgery (see note pg 72).

PN- A client may be hypersensitive to touch & pain. Deep or aggressive massage may irritate inflamed joints & tissues, leading to increased pain or swelling, particularly during flare-ups. Talk with clients about their needs.

Suggested Questions: Are you on any medications for it currently? Are you doing other self care such as activities to stay active?

Symptoms

- Joint pain/sensitivity
- Reduced ROM
- Inflammation

Contraindications

- Deep Tissue specifically around joints
- Cold Therapy

SEVER'S DISEASE

This is an overuse injury, specifically, inflammation to the growth plate in the heel. This is more common in active children. It's best to avoid the Achille's due to the inflammation. Local contraindication.

Suggested Questions: When do you notice the pain? Is it worse when you're playing or exercising? Does heat or ice help with the pain?

Symptoms

- Heel pain
- Tenderness on the back of the heel
- Client may have a difficult walking or putting all their body weight on affected leg

Contraindication

- Achilles tendon until cleared by PCP

SCIATICA

Sciatica refers to pain, numbness, or tingling radiating along the path of the sciatic nerve, which extends from the lower back, through the buttocks, & down the back of each leg to the foot. It is typically caused by nerve compression or irritation, most commonly from a Herniated Disc(see note pg 63), Bone Spur(see note 28),or Spinal Stenosis (see note 110).

PN- This is a very common pathology however it's also a very common self diagnosed one. Sciatica is pain referred to the back of the back of leg if the client complains of pain on the side of the leg, it's not Sciatica.

Symptoms

- Radiating pain from glute to foot
- Muscle weakness
- Pins & Needles feeling down leg

SCLERODERMA (SYSTEMIC SCLEROSIS)

A chronic autoimmune disease that causes the skin & connective tissues to become thick & hard. It occurs when the body's immune system mistakenly attacks its tissues, leading to fibrosis (scarring) & thickening of the skin &, in some cases, internal organs like the heart, lungs, or kidneys. The skin may become tight, fragile, or more sensitive, so deep tissue massage or strong pressure may cause discomfort or damage to the skin. Inflammatory or painful joints & muscles may become aggravated by massage if not performed gently.

Symptoms

- Muscle twisting or spasms
- Abnormal postures
- Tremors or jerking movements
- Difficulty with motor control
- Voice or speech changes

Contraindications

- Deep Tissue
- Gua sha
- Cupping

SEIZURE DISORDERS

A seizure involves involuntary movements, loss of consciousness, & shaking. If someone is having a seizure, it's crucial to gently position them onto their side to ensure their safety. Epilepsy is one of the most common seizure disorders, with 150,000 new diagnosies in the U.S. each year. Have a plan with your client before the session. Discuss what they need in case they experience a seizure during the massage to ensure their safety. Never massage while a client is actively having a seizure. After a seizure, clients may need extra time to get up from the table, as they are more prone to lightheadedness & dizziness.

Suggested Questions: How long has it been since you've been diagnosed? What does a typical seizure episode look like for you? *(This is critical so you can identify if something unusual occurs & call 911 if needed.)*

Symptoms

- Involuntary shaking
- Loss of consciousness
- Lightheaded/dizziness

SEBORRHEIC KERATOSIS

Common skin growth. Non-cancerous. Can be tan, brown, black, or white, & are usually round or oval. They can have a wax or scaly texture. Massage carries no risk as long as the client isn't bleeding or irritated.

PN- Be aware if it does change between sessions tell the client to see a Dermatologist.

Symptoms

- Raised skin lesions
- Color variation
- "Stuck-on" appearance
- Round or oval shape

SHIN SPLINTS (MTSS)

Medial tibial stress syndrome is an injury most commonly associated with shin splints. This occurs when there is overuse or repetitive stress on the shinbone (tibia) and the tissues attaching muscles to the bone. This leads to inflammation and pain along the inner part of the lower leg. REMEMBER (SHARP). Not appropriate to massage before out of the acute stage (24-48hrs) & getting cleared with a PCP.

Symptoms

- Pain Along the Shinbone
- Swelling
- Pain During Activity

Contraindication

- Local (if SHARP is present)

SINUSITIS

Inflammation or infection of the sinuses, typically caused by a cold or allergies, leading to symptoms like facial pain, nasal congestion, & headache.

Do NOT MASSAGE clients until they have been cleared by PCP

Symptoms

- Fever
- Nasal congestion
- Cough
- Flu like symptoms

Contraindication

- DO NOT MASSAGE until cleared by PCP

SPONDYLOLISTHESIS

A condition in which a structural problem in the lumbar spine allows one or more vertebral bodies to slip anteriorly. There are many different types. *PN-* Understanding more specifics will better help with your sessions. What are there goals for massage therapy?

- **Congenital:** Present at birth due to spinal malformation.
- **Isthmic:** Caused by a stress fracture in a vertebra, often seen in athletes.
- **Degenerative:** Due to aging & wear-&-tear on spinal joints & discs.
- **Traumatic:** Caused by direct injury to the spine.
- **Pathologic:** Linked to diseases like Osteoporosis (*see note*) or cancer.

Symptoms
- Pain may be targeted in the low back/radiating pain
- Muscle weakness
- Numbness or tingling

Contraindications (general)
- Deep Tissue on lumbar spine
- Back stretches

SPINAL STENOSIS

This is when there's narrowing of the spinal column, putting pressure on the spinal cord & nerve roots. Targets the curves in the spine, neck & lower back.

PN- Open communication is necessary for client's comfort in position on table.

Suggested Questions: Are there any ROM or activities that are painful to do? Do you wear any prescribed braces?

Symptoms

- Numbness/tingling (neck, back arms & legs)
- Difficulty Balancing
- Loss of bladder control

SPONDYLOSIS

A form of degenerative arthritis, (see note pg 22) involving age-related changes of the cervical vertebrae, and cartilage. The main risk for clients with spondylosis is careless positioning on the table. Some positions may exacerbate symptoms.

Symptoms
- Stiffness/pain
- Reduced ROM

SUNBURN

A skin inflammation caused by overexposure to ultraviolet (UV) radiation, typically from the sun or tanning devices. It presents as red, painful skin that may peel as it heals.

PN-Most of the time clients will have sunburns on their limbs & face due to lack of sun protection. The unaffected skin can be massaged like normal.

Symptoms

- Redness of skin
- Hot to the touch
- Peeling of the Skin

Contraindication

- Local

TARSAL TUNNEL SYNDROME

TTS is caused by compression of the posterior tibial nerve in the tarsal tunnel, located behind the medial malleolus (ankle).

PN- If the nerve is compressed or inflamed, the client may not have full feeling of that area.

Suggested Questions: How long has it been since your diagnosis? Are you doing any kind of self care that helps mitigate the pain? Are you seeing a PT? Is there any specific time or activity that makes this flair up?

Symptoms

- Burning
- Tingling
- Shooting pain in the foot or ankle
- Numbness in the sole of the foot

Contraindication

- Local

TATTOOS (NEW)

New tattoos are a local contraindication. A fresh tattoo is an open wound where ink is deposited into the dermis layer of the skin. It requires proper aftercare to heal & avoid complications such as infection. Tattoos past the healing stage (about one month) can be massaged as normal.

Contraindication
- Local

TENNIS ELBOW & GOLF ELBOW

Both conditions involve inflammation or degeneration of the tendons where they attach to the elbow, caused by overuse or repetitive strain. *PN-* To remember which one is which tennis L- Ladies Golf Medial-Men (Lateral Epicondylitis)(Medial Epicondylitis)

Symptoms
- Pain & tenderness on the outer elbow/ also radiating pain to forearm
- Weak grip strength, especially during lifting or gripping.

Contraindication
- Local until cleared by PCP

TENDINOPATHIES

Tendinopathy is usually a type of overuse injury, where the tendon is repeatedly strained until tiny tears form. It commonly affects the shoulder, wrist, knee, shin, & heel. Acute injuries are a local contraindication.

Suggested Questions: Are you doing anything at home for self care? Are you in PT?

Symptoms

- Crepitus
- Gradual Onset
- Warmth or Redness

Contraindication

- Local (acute stage)

TEMPOROMANDIBULAR JOINT (TMJ)

Common problems around the jaw are usually associated with some combination of malocclusion (abnormal teeth alignment) grinding teeth & loose ligaments surrounding the jaw. It is important to have an accurate diagnosis of jaw pain because some of the disorders that mimic TMJ disorders may contraindicate MT in some cases.

PN- If trained intraoral work may help clients symptoms.

Symptoms

- Jaw Pain or Tenderness
- Clicking or Popping Sounds
- Headaches or Migraines
- Ear aches/ pain or ringing

THORACIC OUTLET SYNDROME

A group of conditions involving neurovascular entrapments in the neck or anterior shoulder region. In some cases, Thoracic Outlet Syndrome may be linked to anatomical variations, which cannot be altered through massage therapy.

PN- For this pathology, the primary focus should be on mitigating pain, understanding that the approach may vary from other conditions. When collaborating as part of a comprehensive wellness team, the goal is to work together to support the client's overall well-being.

Symptoms

- Numbness tingling down arm to fingers
- Chronic Pain

TUBERCULOSIS

This is a very serious bacterial infection that targets the lungs. Is contagious, airborne. Do NOT MASSAGE clients until they have been cleared by PCP

Symptoms

- Flu like symptoms
- Chest pain
- Coughing up blood

Contraindication

- DO NOT MASSAGE until cleared by PCP

VESTIBULAR BALANCE DISORDERS

(VBDs) are a group of conditions that can cause debilitating vertigo that may last anywhere from a few seconds to many hours.

PN- Getting up & down from the table. These clients are prone to dizzy spells. acupressure technique may be used however if it makes the client feel vertigo don't use the technique a craniosacral session is also recommended.

Suggested Questions: Are you taking any medications for the vertigo?

Symptoms

- Vertigo
- Dizziness
- Nausea or Vomiting

VITILIGO

This is a chronic skin condition characterized by the loss of pigment (melanin) in certain areas of the skin, resulting in white or depigmented patches.

PN-Micheal Jackson had this condition. This is a NON contagious condition. No coundraindications.

Symptoms

- White or Depigmented patches on skin
- Skin sensitvity

WARTS

They are small, rough, & usually benign growths on the skin. Non-contagious. They can be anywhere on the body but most common is on the hands, arms & face.

PN- If you are concerned a wart may be infected, talk with your client to see a PCP. Contraindications are only over warts. Rest if the body can be massaged like normal.

Symptoms

- Small, grainy bumps
- Raised or flat
- Flesh-colored or slightly darker

Contraindications local

- Cupping
- Gua sha

WHIPLASH

Cervical spine acceleration-deceleration is used to explain the combination of injuries. A client with recent neck trauma MUST be cleared by PCP. Whiplash pain doesn't come to light until days after the accident.

PN- Neuromuscular MT are good to consult. PT would be also good to work with since a client may have PT after a serious accident.

Suggested Questions: Are you taking any medications? How did the accident occur?

Symptoms

- Neck pain
- Limited ROM
- Muscle spasms
- Shoulder pain

Contraindication

- DO NOT MASSAGE until cleared by PCP

ZOSTER (SHINGLES)

Shingles, or *(Herpes Zoster)*, is a viral infection of the same virus that causes chickenpox. After a person recovers from chickenpox, the virus remains dormant in nerve tissues & can reactivate later in life, leading to shingles. Clients with shingles will have painfull blistering rash, burning tingling or itching over affected area. DO NOT massage a client with active shingles.

Symptoms

- Pain & tingling
- Rash development
- Blisters

Contraindication

- DO NOT MASSAGE until cleared by PCP

MEDICATIONS TO UNDERSTAND WHAT QUESTIONS TO ASK

NSAIDs Non-Steroidal Anti-Inflammatory drugs used for pain relief inflammation and fever- ibuprofen: advil; motrin: naproxen; aleve:aspirin

Opioids used for pain relieving targets the nervous system- Hydrocodone, Oxycodone, Morphine, Ultram (Tramadol)- If a client is on this medication before massage do NOT overwork or go deep with the client. Can alway reschedule due to the client not having a full feeling of pain reception.

Anticoagulants used as blood thinners- Warfarin-(Coumadin) Apixaban(eliquis) Clopidogrel(Plavix)

ALL used to prevent blood clots- Clients on these medications have an increased risk of bleeding, bruising or internal bleeding. **DO NOT** use DT or any other aggressive techniques including cupping & Gua sha on the skin. Antihypertensives (blood pressure) Beta-blockers metoprolol atenolol.

Suggested Question: Have they been cleared for massage by a doctor if they are taking opioids after major surgeries or accidents.

ACE inhibitors used for hypertension- lisinopril,(generic) enalapril. (generic) This increases the risk of the client being dizzy & dehydrated. Allow more time to get up & down from the table.

Calcium Channel Blockers(CCB's) used to relax blood vessels and reduce blood pressure- amlodipine(Norvasc) Felodipine(Plendil) Nicardipine (cardene)

Cholesterol-lowering Statins Atorvastatin (Lipitor), Simvastatin(Zocor)

PN- Our job isn't to interrogate our clients **EVER**! Remember, this may take time to gather from a client who isn't comfortable speaking of undergoing treatment. This section is simply to understand what these treatments do to the body & what techniques may be better for that client at that time.

HORMONE FERTILITY TREATMENT

Hormone fertility treatment is used in many different cases for all kinds of different reasons. Physical effects include bloating or abdominal pain.

- Tenderness to Breasts
- Headaches/Fatigue
- Weight fluctuations
- Changes in skin (extra sensitivity)
- Mood swings
- A client may be more sensitive to smells from emollients or aromatherapy

Suggested Questions:
- Have you been cleared for massage due to the increased risk of blood clots ?
- How long have they been going through treatments?
- What side effects do they feel are impacting their life most?

HRT for Menopause:
- This treatment is to help manage menopause symptoms, hot flashes, mood swings, & bone density loss
- Menopause can start for women between 45-55 last for about a year

Symptoms

- Fluid retention
- Breast tenderness
- Skin Sensitivities/more prone to bruising

Suggested Questions: How long have they been experiencing symptoms? Have you seen your dr? What would you like to get out of the massage today?

Weight LOSS/Metabolic management- loose skin, surgical scars. Suggested technique, lymphatic.

CORTICOSTEROID Therapy- It's a shot for pain (eg. carpal tunnel syndrome) that is used for treatment so that surgery can be postponed.

DIALYSIS- Cardiac treatments: post surgery recovery; bypass stents. Clients may have muscle soreness & fatigue from healing. Pacemakers or defibrillators: cautious around the chest scarring, also ask if the client is comfortable being on their stomach for an extended amount of time.

COSMETIC or Dermatological treatments- Botox fillers: ask where it is (client may use for chronic headaches) avoid pressure on or near the injection site for 24-48 hours.

Laser hair removal or micro-needling- avoid massage on treated areas until fully healed.

Organ transplant recovery- Super cautious with DT on client. Increased risk of bruising. Clients are more likely to obtain an infection. Client should be cleared by PCP for massage therapy.

Circulatory & Immune Systems

These cancers involve treatments that typically affect blood, lymph nodes, & the immune system.

- Cancer Types:
- Leukemia (Blood cancer)
- Lymphoma (Lymphatic system cancer)

Common Treatments:

Chemotherapy-Kills rapidly dividing cells; also affects healthy blood cells, leading to immune suppression, anemia, & fatigue.

Bone Marrow Transplant-May be used to restore healthy blood cells after chemotherapy.

Radiation-Targets specific areas, often to destroy lymphatic cancer or blood cancer cells.

Digestive & Metabolic Systems

These cancers affect organs involved in digestion & metabolism, such as the liver, pancreas, & gastrointestinal tract.

Cancer Types:

- Liver Cancer
- Pancreatic Cancer
- Colorectal Cancer

Common Treatments

Chemotherapy-Often used for metastatic or advanced cancers, but can also damage healthy cells in the digestive system.

Surgery-Often involves removal of a portion of the liver, pancreas, or colon.

Radiation-Used to shrink tumors in the digestive organs.

Targeted Therapy-Works on specific pathways in cancer cells to reduce growth.

System Impacts:

- Nausea, vomiting, & diarrhea (due to chemotherapy or radiation).
- Fatigue (from treatment side effects).
- Weight loss & digestive issues (especially after surgery or removal of organs).
- Liver dysfunction (from liver cancer treatments, which can affect metabolism).
- Hormonal & Reproductive Systems

Cancers in these areas often require hormonal therapies or treatments that disrupt hormone production.

Cancer Types:

- Breast Cancer
- Prostate Cancer
- Ovarian Cancer

Common Treatments

Hormonal Therapy: Used for hormone-sensitive cancers (e.g., estrogen-receptor-positive breast cancer) to block or reduce hormone production.

Surgery: Removal of reproductive organs

Chemotherapy: Targets rapidly dividing cells impacts healthy reproductive cells.

Radiation: Often localized to the affected area, such as the breast or prostate.

System Impacts:

- Fatigue (from chemotherapy & hormonal treatments).
- Hot flashes & night sweats (from hormonal therapy, especially for breast or prostate cancer).
- Decreased libido & fertility issues (due to hormone therapy or surgery).
- Bone density loss (from hormone-blocking treatments).

Respiratory System

Lung cancer treatments focus on the lungs & surrounding structures, which can impact breathing & circulation.

Cancer Types:

- Lung Cancer

Common Treatments:

Surgery: Removal of part or all of a lung.

Chemotherapy & Radiation: Used to shrink tumors & destroy cancer cells.

Targeted Therapy & Immunotherapy: Used for specific genetic mutations or to boost the immune response against cancer cells.

System Impacts:

- Shortness of breath (due to surgery or damage from cancer or radiation).
- Fatigue (due to treatment & poor oxygenation).
- Chest pain (post-surgery or due to the tumor pressing on nearby structures).
- Lymphedema (especially after lymph node removal in the chest area).

Skin & Soft Tissue

Skin cancer treatments often involve surgery or radiation that affects the skin's integrity & healing.

Cancer Types:

- Skin Cancer (eg. Melanoma)

Common Treatments:

Surgery: Removal of cancerous skin lesions.

Radiation: Targets cancerous skin cells, especially if surgery is not an option.

Topical Chemotherapy: Applied directly to the skin

Immunotherapy: Used for advanced melanoma.

System Impacts:

- Skin sensitivity & irritation (from radiation or surgery).
- Wound healing issues (especially after surgery or radiation).
- Fatigue (due to systemic treatments like immunotherapy).

Urinary & Excretory Systems

These cancers impact the kidneys, bladder, & related systems, often requiring surgical or systemic interventions.

Cancer Types:

- Bladder Cancer
- Kidney Cancer

Common Treatments:

Surgery: Removal of part or all of the bladder or kidney.

Chemotherapy: Used for advanced cases or metastasis.

Immunotherapy & Targeted Therapy: Used for specific types of bladder or kidney cancers.

System Impacts:

- Fatigue (due to chemotherapy & surgery).
- Urinary issues (difficulty urinating or frequent urination after bladder surgery).
- Lymphedema (in the legs after lymph node removal in pelvic cancers).

Summary: Cancer Treatment & Systemic Impacts

- Circulatory & Immune Systems: Leukemia & lymphoma treatment impact blood cells, leading to immune suppression, fatigue, & bruising.
- Digestive & Metabolic Systems: Liver, pancreatic, & colorectal cancer treatments lead to nausea, weight loss, fatigue, & digestive problems.
- Hormonal & Reproductive Systems: Breast, prostate, & ovarian cancer treatments disrupt hormones, causing fatigue, hot flashes, & bone density loss.
- Respiratory System: Lung cancer treatments cause shortness of breath, fatigue, & chest pain.
- Skin & Soft Tissue: Skin cancer treatments lead to skin sensitivity & wound healing issues.
- Urinary & Excretory Systems: Bladder & kidney cancer treatments can result in urinary problems & fatigue.

Clients in Addiction Recovery

May experience, sensitivity to touch & Overstimulation

Reason: Individuals in recovery may have heightened sensitivity to touch or overstimulation, especially if they have a history of physical or emotional trauma.

Massage Consideration: Be mindful of pressure & start with lighter techniques. Always ask for feedback during the session & adjust accordingly.

Withdrawal Symptoms:

- Reason: Depending on the severity of the addiction, withdrawal symptoms can include muscle aches, tension, anxiety, & fatigue. These symptoms may still be present even after a person has begun recovery.

- Massage Consideration: Some techniques may exacerbate withdrawal symptoms, especially if the individual is still experiencing physical discomfort or has yet to stabilize their nervous system. Gentle strokes & relaxation techniques can be more appropriate during early recovery stages.

Circulatory & Heart Issues:

- Reason: Long-term substance abuse (e.g., stimulants like methamphetamine, or opioids) can affect the cardiovascular system, causing heart rate irregularities, high blood pressure, or circulatory problems.

- Massage Consideration: Be cautious when performing techniques that affect circulation, such as deep tissue work, especially around the chest & neck area. Monitor blood pressure & heart rate, & avoid areas where there may be known cardiovascular issues.

Lymphatic System:

- Drugs can affect the liver, kidneys, & lymphatic system, all of which play a role in detoxification.
- Massage Consideration: Techniques that promote lymphatic drainage or gentle circulatory stimulation can help support detoxification, but be aware of how the client reacts to these techniques. Overly intense manipulation may trigger discomfort or fatigue.

Emotional & Psychological Triggers:

- Reason: Recovery from addiction often comes with emotional challenges, such as depression, anxiety, or even post-traumatic stress disorder (PTSD), especially if the addiction was a coping mechanism for past trauma.
- Massage Consideration: Creating a safe & supportive environment is crucial. Talk to the client about any emotional triggers that might arise during a session. Some individuals may experience emotional release during a massage, so be prepared to offer a calming presence &, if needed, refer to a mental health professional for support.

Skin Sensitivity & Healing:

- Reason: Certain drugs, especially stimulants like methamphetamine, can affect the skin, leading to conditions such as skin lesions, bruising, or scarring.
- Massage Consideration: Be gentle in areas where there might be healing wounds or scars, & avoid deep pressure on those areas. Keep the client's comfort in mind when addressing any known skin conditions.

Medication Interactions:

- Reason: Individuals in recovery are often prescribed medications for pain management, anxiety, or other conditions related to recovery. These medications can affect muscle tone, blood pressure, or nervous system function.
- Massage Consideration: Be aware of common medications, such as benzodiazepines, opioid substitutes (e.g., methadone, buprenorphine), & antidepressants. These medications can cause sedation or affect muscle tone, so adjust techniques accordingly (e.g., avoiding deep pressure or heat modalities if the client is on sedatives)

ELDERLY CARE

Parkinson's- Parkinson's disease is a progressive neurodegenerative disorder that affects movement. It occurs when nerve cells in the brain, particularly those producing dopamine, are damaged or die. This leads to issues with movement control, balance, & coordination. *PN-* A very well-known celebrity Muhammad Ali had Parkinsons' later in life.

Symptoms

- Tremors
- Bradykinesia (Slowness of Movement)
- Muscle stiffness
- Postural Instability
- Speech changes (monotone voice)
- swallowing difficulties
- sometimes cognitive changes or depression

Clients treatment may include

- Medications Levodopa: The most common medication, which the brain converts into dopamine.
- Surgical Procedure Deep Brain Stimulation (DBS): A procedure that involves implanting electrodes into the brain to regulate abnormal brain activity.
- Physical Therapy: Focuses on improving mobility, balance, & coordination through targeted exercises.
- **Suggested Questions**: How long have you been diagnosed? Have you tried any kind of treatment that's worked so far? What are your goals for seeing an MT?

***Hemiplegia*-**(*Stroke recovery*)- Hemiplegia is a condition where one side of the body becomes paralyzed, often because of a stroke. A stroke happens when the blood flow to part of the brain is blocked or reduced, causing brain cells to die & leading to problems with movement, speech, & other body functions. Stroke Recovery involves the process of rehabilitation (PT) following a stroke, aiming to restore function & improve the quality of life for individuals affected by the condition. Recovery time varies depending on how severe the stroke was.

Symptoms

- Paralysis
- Muscle weakness
- Impaired coronation & balance
- Stiff muscles on the affected side
- Numbness
- Speech & swallowing problems

Medications to note:

- Antiplatelet(Helps prevent blood clots from forming, preventing another stroke)
- Anticoagulants (Blood Thinners)
- Meds to control blood pressure

Suggested Questions: How long has it been since the incident? Are you seeing a Physical therapist currently? What would you like to get out of the massage? Has your doctor made sure your blood clots are gone? *PN-* I wouldn't recommend cupping or Gua sha, especially on older clients whose skin is more fragile

SUPPLEMENT BENEFITS

(Not for us to prescribe them to clients! For us to understand their purpose within the body.)

1. B-12

Benefits:

- Supports nerve health- Essential for maintaining the myelin sheath, which protects nerves and ensures efficient signal transmission.
- Boosts Energy & red blood cell production- Helps prevent fatigue by aiding in the fomation of healthy red blood cells,improvinf oxegen delivery to muscles and tissues.
- Reduces muscle weakness & tingling- Helps prevent symtoms like muscle weakness, numbness and tingling.

2. Calcium

Benefits:

- Bone health: Calcium is essential for maintaining strong bones & preventing osteoporosis & fractures, especially in aging adults.
- Muscle function: Helps with muscle contraction & relaxation, reducing the risk of muscle cramps & tension.

3. Vitamin C

Benefits:

- Antioxidant protection: Vitamin C is an antioxidant that helps fight damage in the body & supports healthy tissue repair.
- Immune system support
- Skin health

4. Vitamin D

Benefits:

- Bone health: Vitamin D helps the body absorb calcium, which is important for strong bones & joint health
- Immune support
- Mood regulation

5. Iron

Benefits:

- Oxygen transport: Iron is crucial for the production of hemoglobin, which carries oxygen in the blood. It can help improve energy levels & reduce fatigue in clients with iron-deficiency anemia.

6. Magnesium

Benefits:

- Muscle relaxation: Magnesium plays a critical role in muscle function & relaxation. It can help alleviate muscle cramps, tension, & fibromyalgia pain.
- Nervous system support
- Bone health: It helps with calcium absorption, supporting strong bones & joints

7. Omega-3 Fatty Acids (Fish Oil or Flaxseed Oil)

Benefits:

- Anti-inflammatory: Omega-3 fatty acids are known for reducing systemic inflammation & are commonly used to help manage conditions like arthritis, cardiovascular disease, & autoimmune disorders.
- Joint health
- Heart health: They can lower triglyceride levels & reduce the risk of heart disease.
- Cognitive support

8. Probiotics

Benefits:

- Gut health: Probiotics are beneficial bacteria that support a healthy gut microbiome, which can improve digestion, immune function, & skin health.
- Mental health benefits
- Anti-inflammatory effects: Can help reduce systemic inflammation & may be beneficial for conditions like irritable bowel syndrome (IBS)

9. Turmeric (Curcumin)

Benefits:

- Anti-inflammatory properties: Normally used to reduce inflammation, which can help with conditions like arthritis, muscle soreness, & joint pain.
- Digestive support: It may help improve digestion & reduce bloating or indigestion.

10. Zinc

Benefits:

- Immune support: Zinc is crucial for the proper functioning of the immune system & can help fight off infections & support wound healing.
- Skin health: It supports healthy skin & can help manage acne, eczema, & other skin conditions.
- Antioxidant properties: Zinc is an antioxidant & supports the body's defense against oxidative stress.

www.ingramcontent.com/pod-product-compliance
Lightning Source LLC
Chambersburg PA
CBHW070633030426
42337CB00020B/3999